Don't Inflict Emotional Torture

Change your Eating Habits

And Live a Healthy Lifestyle

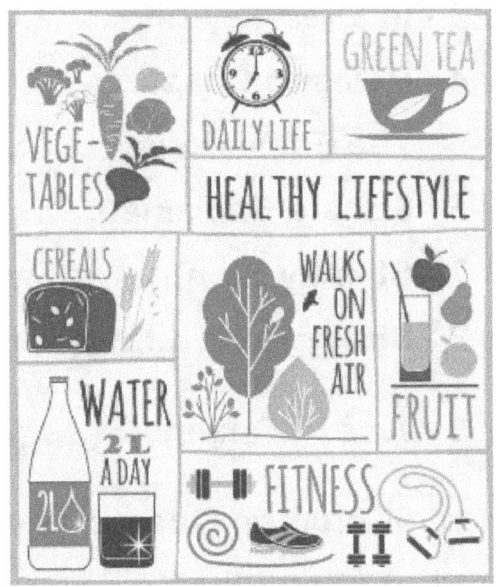

By: Sue Feldman (Nutritionist)

Medical Disclaimer:

The information in this book is not intended to replace a 1-on-1 relationship with a qualified medical professional and it is not intended as medical advice. It is intended as a sharing of knowledge and information. I encourage you to make your own health core decisions based upon your research and in partnership with your doctor. You know your body and how it feels; sometimes a sore in your side might be more than a pulled muscle. So, taking a pain killer tablet might help the pain but not cure the underlining reason why you got the pain in the first place. Self-diagnose, is the first step, know thy self. You can become a healthier, happier and more successful person by making a few simple changes to your lifestyle and eating habits.

This publication is part of a series of products and publications.

Introduction – My story

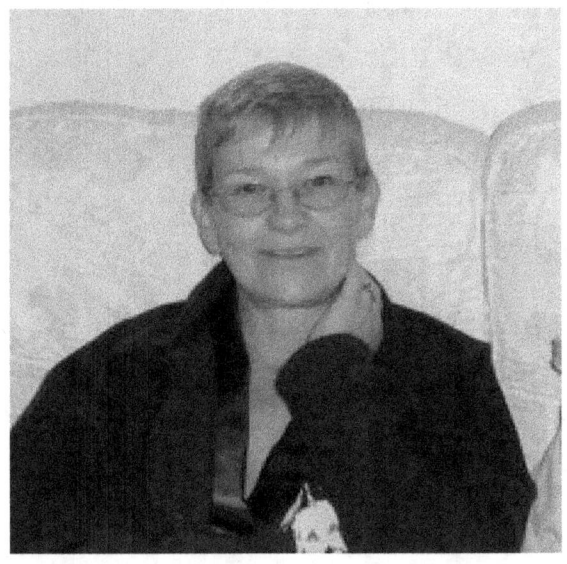

I have been a Nutritionist since 1998 and been interested in health issues all my life. I believe that we need to take extra vitamins and minerals supplements, as the fresh food we eat today is not as healthy as in our grandparents' days; our soil has been depleted of minerals from mass production.

I have to say this: that it's your body and if something does not feel right get to the bottom of it - go for blood tests or even xrays to get answers. General Practitioners - GP's, only study about 3 to 5% of nutrition in all the years they study to become doctors. You can become a healthier, happier and more successful person by making a few simple changes to your eating habits and lifestyle.

Don't be the person who misses out on the opportunities in life because you don't understand the necessary principles of healthy living. Be the kind of person others marvel at. Be the kind of person other people see and say, "I don't know how you stay and look so good". Be the kind of person who acts.

The information in this book is intended as a sharing of knowledge and information. I encourage you to make your own health core decisions.

My health has been a consistent feature in my life. Since I was a kid, what I remember, is that my father was ill for most of my childhood. I used to nurse him and help whenever I could. He was in and out of hospital, so I never knew if he would be home when I got back from school.

To cut a long story short, he suffered from diabetics, heart problems (9 coronaries) and high cholesterol, ate lots of very rich and unhealthy foods, and smoked like a trouper.

He ended up getting gangrene on his toes and had to have his legs, from his knees down, amputated. At the time of the first operation, the surgeon started on his better leg, but my dad had a heart attack on the operation table, so they did not amputate both legs.

They had to stop and send him home with only completing half of the removal. He lived another 4 years with his bad leg then went for the second operation and died on the table. I was 11 years old!

I also have a sister who lives with a weight problem and since she was 6 months old, she was put on diet. I vowed as a kid that I would never be fat, and I have lived my whole life making sure mentally and physically that I would be slim and trim. My whole family are on the larger size of their idea weight, but not me.

So, I decided to study as much as possible about Health. Then in 1998 I completed a course in a creditable manner and furnished satisfactory evidence of proficiency in Nutritional Therapy and have been entered upon the Register of the Complementary Health Studies Centre.

Hence writing this book to share what I know with others, so that they can become better and healthier and live a happy lifestyle.

Right Attitude
+ Right Mindset
+ Right Foods
+ Right Supplements
+ Right Exercise
_____
Healthy Lifestyle

Chapter 1

Changing Your Eating Habits

This is not about going on a 'diet' to lose a few kilos or pounds; which I am sure you have tried in the past. You decide on a diet plan, stick with it for a couple of weeks or a month, and maybe get to your goal weight. Then you go back to your 'normal eating habits'. So, what happens then – wham, bang, and crash you are back to where you were before, or even bigger! Many have called this 'The Yo-Yo dieter'!

Therefore, don't go on a Diet – change your mind-set and eating habits!

Think of the word 'Diet' as:

Don't **I**nflict **E**motional **T**orture and don't **DIE** for i**T**

Don't inflict emotional torture on your body and mind trying to get it healthy, as soon as you think or someone says you need to go on a 'diet' your mind rebels and all of a sudden you are craving (a killer crave like an addiction) for everything that you are *not supposed* to eat. Therefore, <u>*don't die for it.*</u> Simply change to a healthy eating plan. Notice what you eat because 'you *are* what you eat'.

Remember this: - "If you always do what you always did, you'll always get what you always got".

Typically, when a person thinks of changing their eating habits, they reflect on being obsessive with food. The reality is that the two could be completely opposite. Provided you are trying to live a healthy lifestyle, there are a few measures you must make in order to reach your objectives.

Today the biggest problem is that 'fat' has been taken out of some foods, but to preserve it the companies had to add 'sugar'. Sugar is poison to your body – it destroys your teeth, it makes you fat, and it causes untold diseases and dis-ease. Sugar does not give you energy in the long run, it's gives you a false high, then when it is burnt off you need another fix (of sugar). So, sugar is really an addiction - so if you need energy have protein instead, as it is the fuel for your body.

Your life should be run like a fancy car – when people pay for an expensive car they look after it. It is done by putting in the right gas or petrol, clean water and good oil. One does not buy a car to stand in the garage just to look pretty; it needs to be driven (exercised). And of course, it is kept clean and the outside is waxed to keep it shiny, like new.

So why do we not look after our body like that? The body needs the right gas (called proteins), clean water and good oil or fats. And our body needs to be cleansed (a Detox program, see chapter 11) and the wax is doing exercises or just being active.

Following are some tips to push you to begin:

-- *Thinking and seeing yourself as slim and healthy*

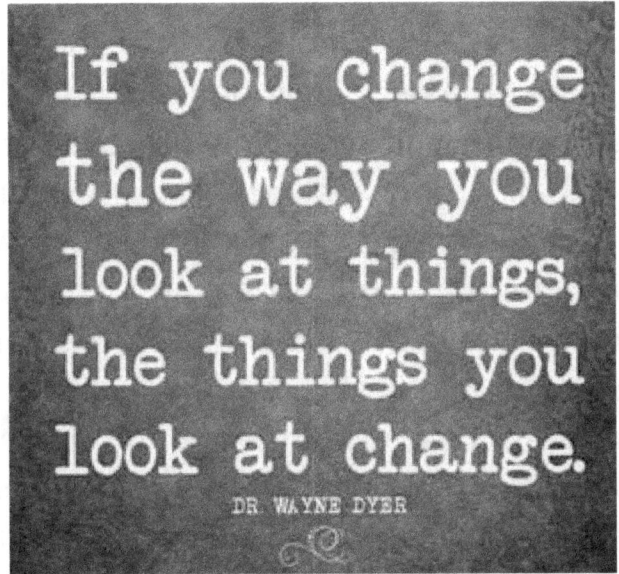

If you change the way you look at things, the things you look at change.

DR. WAYNE DYER

The biggest mistake that anyone could experience when attempting to change their eating habits is falling short with this vital tip. If you choose to not observe yourself as slim and healthy, it will be difficult. That is how dependent it is to change your eating habits - is on thinking and seeing yourself as slim and healthy.

In case you are curious how to think and see yourself as slim and healthy, then don't weigh yourself daily. If you are overweight use a pair of jeans or a belt to measure if you have lost any weight along the way of eating the right kind of healthy foods. Love yourself and think yourself slim! Power of using your mind! Use energy to focus on your ideal body, remember if you focus on the negative that's what you will get, so see and believe what you want and eventually you will get it. The ideal body for you!

-- Making choices that are right for you and not conforming to others

> # Making choices isn't always easy.
> # But, you always have a choice.

Making choices that are right for you and not conforming to others helps you change your eating habits. Understandably, it could be hard to get in the habit of doing it. Begin by making choices that are right and not conforming to what is just dished up every day, and it ought to become force of habit when you change your eating habits.

-- Having healthy eating options

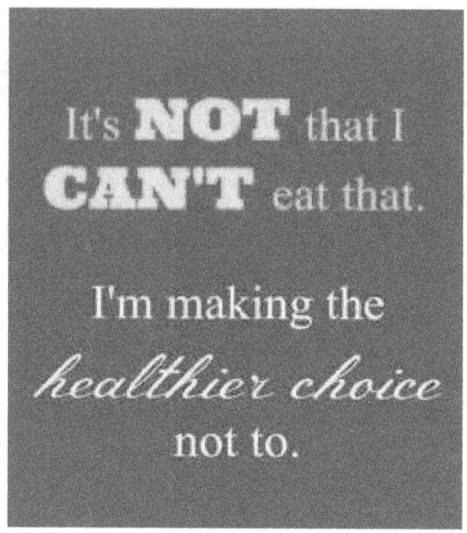

An integral part of the foundation that is necessary to change your eating habits involves having healthy eating options. When you have healthy eating option, it allows you to be in an appropriate mind-set to achieve the utmost goal of changing.

Although we will help you prepare looking at what you eat differently, you initially need to make sure that changing your eating habits is appropriate for you. Looking at what you eat differently is the key, and you must think about it before going forward.

Since you recognize that you are in the right mind-set to change your eating habits, we can examine certain preliminary practices that one would already be doing. Use that opportunity to draw in these practices into your life because it will make preparing to change easier.

One of the best ways to determine whether you will be capable to change is to analyse the day-to-day practices of folks who have already changed their eating habits. You would not need to emulate their accomplishments all at once, as that would be difficult.

Yet, you must be equipped to put forth as much time as they do. Imitate their practices, as they are exactly where you want to be. In addition, reflect on these questions:

Are your eating habits the same as your family (do you all have the same health/weight problems)?

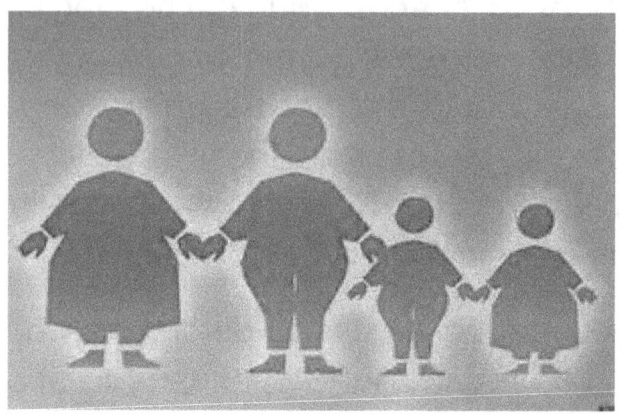

Are you addicted to junk food? (Are all your meals take-outs?)

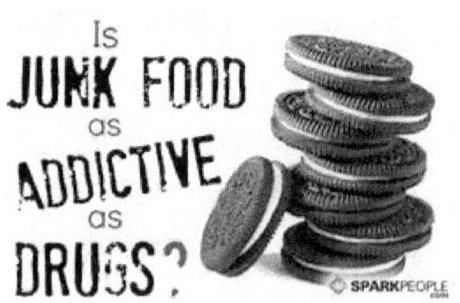

Is your body slowing down with aches and pain?

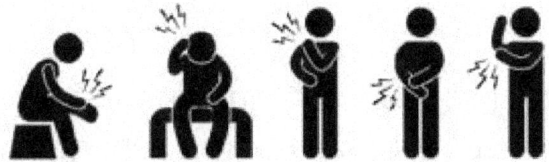

Ideally, you replied positively to these questions. Then probably changing your eating habits is an appropriate activity for you. Congratulations for committing to that initial step forward toward accomplishing your goals by continuing to read!

Changing your eating habits takes heaps of effort invested over time. As you can see, the best way to get equipped for changing your eating habits is to offer yourself the suggested timeframe for your footwork so you can prevail. Do that and changing your eating habits could be much easier.

Chapter 2

Changing Your Eating Habits - A Look Back

Realize that you aren't the first person in the world that has the goal of changing your eating habits. In fact, there are tons of men and women all over that want to look at what they eat differently. The indisputable reality is that only a handful of people will really make the commitment and accomplish it.

Usually the people who do change, do so because of a health issue, like having cancer, or getting diabetes or a heart attack. Changing sooner rather than later before dis-eases set-in is a good idea.

Don't think of being obsessive with food. Eat 3 meals a day, to keep yourself energised. Drink plenty of water when you feel hungry, as water can give you a feeling of being full.

Changing your eating habits necessitates one to be changeable and steadfast. We recognize this. Now we are prepared to analyse the stages recommended with changing your eating habits so we can enjoy our future accomplishments.

If you study others who have done well in changing their eating habits either now or long ago, you will discover one thing in common among the personalities who have done well.

They knew what was recommended before starting, and they appreciated what type of person is likely to prevail. When you recognize what kind of individual is necessary to change, determined and committed, there is not anyone that will block the path between you and your success!

Being entirely focused to change your eating habits requires dedication mentally, along with physically. The number one method to train all around is to have a strong mentality and get mentally prepared.

You should probably take this time to check whether you have the gumption it takes. Do you have a changeable personality? It is a vital part of the formula that everyone who expects to change their eating habits needs, or else looking at what you eat differently will get ridiculously hard, if not unfeasible.

Additionally, make sure you have the drive that changing your eating habits will take. Are your eating habits the same as your family (do you all have the same health/weight problems)? There could be a major difference between contemplating something as a beneficial idea and ultimately doing it. Without a doubt, you'd need a ton of discipline, desire, willpower and determination to move forward.

You've already taken a big step towards being equipped to change your eating habits. Some people botch up for good reason. They simply did not recognize what precisely they were getting themselves into.

Changing your eating habits is that one thing in life that necessitates you to get entirely steadfast and prepared. Through looking forward and making sure you are changeable and beneficial; you would be taking the first step toward preparing.

Also consider that choosing to change is equally important to your health success. Your mind might try to persuade you that changing your eating habits could be rather hard or is probably not worth the effort, but by choosing to change and maintaining concentration on your goal, you will do it! Let's determine how we will now plan for changing your eating habits!

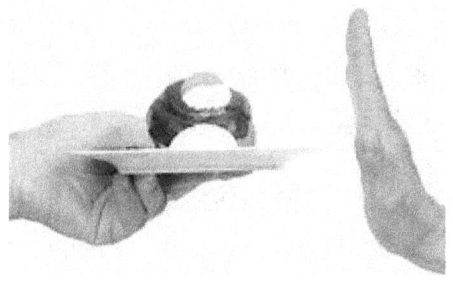

Chapter 3

Changing Your Eating Habits in Everyday Life

During the time you look at what you eat for 1 week, by writing down every morsel that passes your lips, you would discover that changing your eating habits is impacting other aspects of your life. Changing your eating habits is a major lifestyle choice that impacts you in many ways.

Tip: Get my Coulouring Journal and Food Diary from amazon.com to jot everything down that you eat.

Along with looking at your lifestyle, the 3 questions are also looking to analyse your skills and desires. So, if you replied yes to these questions, there is an indication of what is significant to you.

By noting the role these qualities play in your daily life, you are acknowledging the role that changing your eating habits plays in life. Changing what you are eating now is not easy. All rewarding activities necessitate commitment. Changing your eating habits is no exception.

One of the hardest ways to change is if you are a person who enjoys baking. Look at the kind of food you are making, do you use a load of sugar and keep tasting as you are preparing? There are many recipes on the market that do not use sugar, and they are usually diabetic recipes and very delicious too. Most people cannot tell the difference.

Tip: Get my Little Cookbook from amazon.com. Cooking with fruit instead of sugar. Some of the recipes use **STEVIA** sweetener. A study has shown it to be a safe and natural, calorie-free sugar substitute.

Be sure to look at what is necessary before changing. This is exactly what will be impacting in other areas of your life. Making choices that are right for you and not conforming to others, having healthy eating options and thinking and seeing yourself as slim and healthy ought to be acts that overlap looking at what you eat differently. Even though we would be examining this as being specific to changing your eating habits, much of it will change other areas in your life.

The best thing about changing your eating habits is the changeable characteristic that is necessary to succeed which will make its way in all aspects of life. That prepares you to become a more changeable person overall. Anytime you look at what you eat differently, adding some exercise and thinking of your feelings you would be preparing your spirit for what will follow. It is just one of the good things of changing.

One may have a beneficial characteristic to change too. That is one more attribute which impacts your lifestyle. The longer you call on that attribute to look at what you eat differently, the more you will recognize that attribute within unrelated areas of your life.

Changing your eating habits really takes much more out of one than one may think. Changing your eating habits is not only something to try; it is alternatively an entire lifestyle shift. It clearly takes a distinctive set of qualities to change your eating habits successfully and sticking with it.

If you are devoted to completing whatever you begin, having the willpower, changing your eating habits will become another amazing thing which you accomplish in your life. Congratulations with beginning your progression towards a more satisfying healthy lifestyle! Read chapter 11 to give you some ideas on different plans which you could try for yourself.

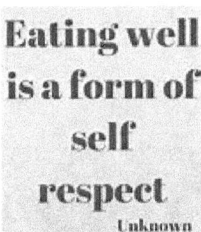

Eating well is a form of self respect
Unknown

Chapter 4

Rules to Consider While Changing Your Eating Habits

As we've recently analysed, changing your eating habits requires quite a bit out of an individual. You should become changeable, beneficial, and determined. Some people may have these traits, but the reality is that preparing for a journey as impacting as changing your eating habits may really strip these traits away from you. Following are a handful of tips you ought to follow that will help your mind nurture these traits.

Preparing yourself for the difficult task of changing your eating habits is time-consuming and you will probably be putting in close to a couple of weeks to prepare. This ought to offer you enough time to ingrain these tips in your regiment.

Just remember 'you are what you eat' so cut out sugar and drink lots of water, this will keep your body hydrated and refreshed. It is one of the outcomes that this guideline will generate. Additionally, you will know what you need to do for you, particularly when the time arrives to forming new eating habits on a regular basis.

Also, remember that people who productively know what is 'healthy' will generally keep a journal or food diary and celebrate milestones. Order your Colouring Journal and Food Diary on Amazon.com It is astonishing how these straightforward guidelines can be such a vital part in a larger goal.

When you see yourself as one who is beneficial, then you may find it relatively simple to incorporate these tips into your regimented process. Additionally, if you choose to keep a journal or food diary and celebrate milestones, then it will foster a feeling of accomplishment as you reach your goals.

Let us not forget our goal of being determined to improve your lifestyle and health. It could need yet another degree of energy during the preparation stage, but it'll be worth it. During the time you are working toward getting into smart routines and getting into good eating habits and drinking water often, you should probably remain with a positive attitude and outlook to living a healthy lifestyle.

Through ascertaining that you maintain this mind-set and willpower, you should dissuade your mind from becoming discouraged and giving up.

Changing how you eat is not being obsessive with food. Even though any person can try to look at what you eat differently, it requires one who's determined and changeable to ultimately accomplish this goal of changing your eating habits.

When making a vow to thoroughly prepare, it is your responsibility to not drop out!

To each of those questions, you if replied yes. This is excellent because we had to determine whether you were determined, changeable and motivated. It is these qualities that will steer you to your success when you finally change your eating habits. So, remember to choose to change, know what is healthy, and be determined to improve your lifestyle and health. Follow the above tips and you will be a healthy and happy person in no time!

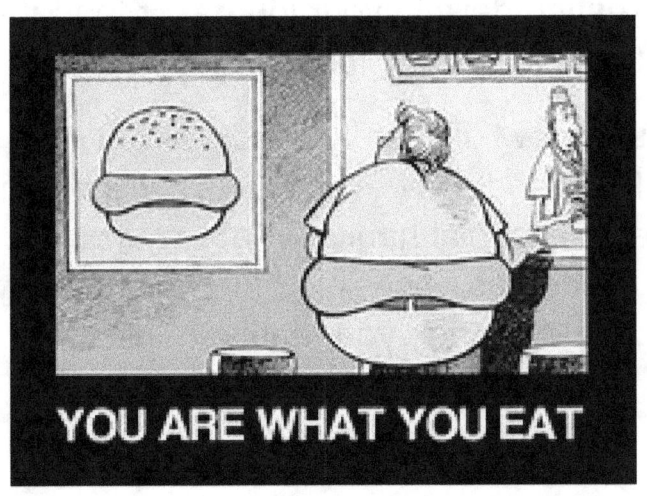

YOU ARE WHAT YOU EAT

Chapter 5

The Easiest Way to Change Your Eating Habits

There are many methods that folks use to change their eating habits. By now, you ought to know that preparation is vital to being successful. Say you are searching for the best method to change your eating habits, and then be sure to offer yourself ample time to find it. Once you do, schedule time to look at what you eat. Usually, 1 week is a standard period to accomplish that goal, by writing and seeing what you are eating daily in your journal or food diary. Is it junk or healthy food?

You're now ultimately ready to get into the task at hand. However, first we will examine a few beneficial habits. That way you are as equipped as possible the moment you decide to change your eating habits.

The steps that you ought to do to prepare to change are: make choices that are right for you and not conforming to others, have healthy eating options and think and see yourself as slim and healthy. Combined these tips make a strong core for your footwork.

Preparing for at least 1 week before you change your eating habits is important and can't be overemphasized. It will show you how and what you are eating that is not healthy in your food journal or diary. It permits you to wholly prepare.

Additionally, it certainly gives you all the beneficial practices necessary for changing. You would discover that choosing to change, knowing what is healthy, and being determined to improve your lifestyle and health will assure that you put forth your best effort possible.

When you disregard these actions, you will forego knowing what you need to do for you, knowing the benefits of healthy eating, and feeling fit and healthy all the time. These results all result from the preparation phase.

With the right scheduling and process, you will certainly be boosting energy, getting into smart routines along with getting into good eating habits and drinking water often. All of these are important to do to change.

The best part of it is: if you can put forth a bit of time into preparing, then it should ultimately get quite simple for you. So, keep from scurrying through any introductory phases. And conclusively, make sure that you are completely ready.

Many folks wrongfully think that it could be hard, or even impossible to become a healthy and vibrant person. Realistically, it just requires one who is changeable, has the willpower, beneficial and determined to ultimately go through the introductory steps.

If you can entirely commit to rejecting short-cuts in the preparation stage and perform all the steps successfully, then you are better positioned to change your eating habits.

The best method to changing your eating habits is to reflect all the steps laid out here. Consequentially, cutting corners is certainly not worth the time and must be avoided while looking at what you eat differently.

You must focus your effort on the first phase of the process as it would make you more productive. The reality is 1 week is not a large amount of time to prepare for such an impacting event as changing your eating habits. So, make the vow to change, put forth the expected amount of time, and you can be changing your eating habits in no time!

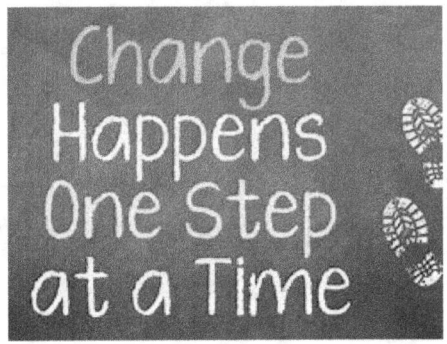

Chapter 6

Sugars Explained

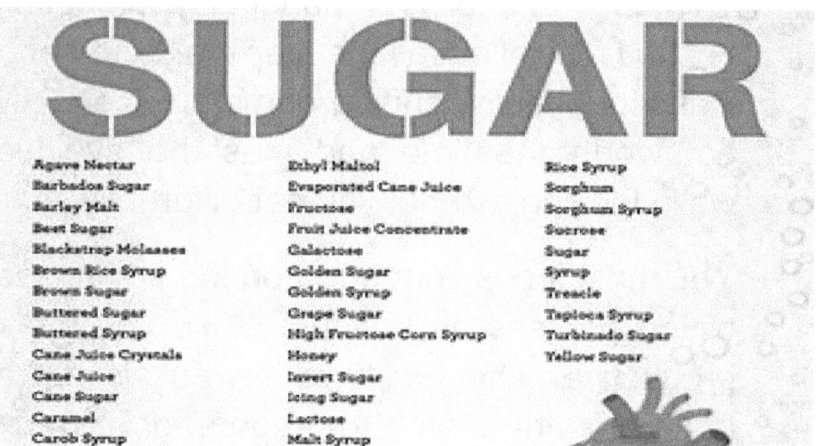

Agave Nectar	Ethyl Maltol	Rice Syrup
Barbados Sugar	Evaporated Cane Juice	Sorghum
Barley Malt	Fructose	Sorghum Syrup
Beet Sugar	Fruit Juice Concentrate	Sucrose
Blackstrap Molasses	Galactose	Sugar
Brown Rice Syrup	Golden Sugar	Syrup
Brown Sugar	Golden Syrup	Treacle
Buttered Sugar	Grape Sugar	Tapioca Syrup
Buttered Syrup	High Fructose Corn Syrup	Turbinado Sugar
Cane Juice Crystals	Honey	Yellow Sugar
Cane Juice	Invert Sugar	
Cane Sugar	Icing Sugar	
Caramel	Lactose	
Carob Syrup	Malt Syrup	

Glucose is the defining standard and has a GI (Glycaemic Index) value of 100. Glucose alone does not taste particularly sweet compared to fructose and sucrose. Glucose is the primary source of energy your body uses, and every cell relies on it to function. When we talk about blood sugar, we are referring to glucose in the blood. When we eat carbohydrates, our body breaks them down into units of glucose. When blood glucose levels rise, cells in the pancreas release insulin, signalling cells to take up glucose from the blood.

Sucrose is crystallized white sugar (white and brown table sugar) produced by the sugar cane plant and can be found in households and foods worldwide. Sucrose is a disaccharide made up of 50% glucose and 50% fructose and is broken down rapidly into its constituent parts.

Due to its glucose content, sucrose has a GI value of 65. As it is made up of glucose and fructose, the latter is metabolized in the liver and holds the same issues as those mentioned for fructose. Due to its glucose content, sucrose does lead to an elevation in blood glucose. Diabetics should therefore be mindful of foods containing sucrose.

Virtually all the fibre, phytochemical, vitamin and mineral content have been removed from white sugar (sucrose). Eating too many carbohydrates, particularly simple sugars, can be harmful to blood sugar control, especially if you are insulin resistant, experience reactive hypoglycaemia or are diabetic. Eating excess sugar can lead to weight gain, which increases the risk of heart disease and type 2 diabetes.

Honey is made up of fructose (40%), glucose (30%), (30%) water and minerals such as iron, calcium, potassium and magnesium. Due to the high level of fructose, honey is sweeter than table sugar. Honey is a high carbohydrate food and has a GI value of 55 (moderate range). Some varieties of honey have a lower GI however, because of fluctuating fructose levels (the more fructose, the lower the GI). Honey is still high in calories and causes increases in blood sugar.

For diabetics or those trying to manage their blood sugar levels, there is no real advantage to substituting sugar for honey as both will ultimately affect blood sugar levels. If you do prefer honey, try to choose a raw variety, which contains more vitamins, enzymes, antioxidants and nutrients than white sugar and use it in moderation.

Fructose is absorbed directly into the bloodstream during digestion and has no impact on insulin production or blood glucose levels.

Consequently, its GI value is much lower, on average around 19. While most diabetics cannot tolerate sucrose, most can tolerate moderate amounts of fruit and fructose without loss of blood sugar control.

__Lactose__ is a sugar found in milk. It is a disaccharide made up of glucose and galactose units. It is broken down into the two parts by an enzyme called lactase. Once broken down, the simple sugars can be absorbed into the bloodstream. Whole milk has a GI value of 41 and is a low GI food. It is broken down slowly and helps to increase the absorption of minerals such as calcium, magnesium and zinc.

Sweeteners

Xylitol, which is a Sugar Alcohol with its low GI value of 7, is broken down slowly, indicating that it **does not cause a spike in blood sugar** or insulin levels and may be helpful in reducing sugar cravings.

Aspartame, Saccharin, Equal, Sweet'N Low are all-Natural Sweeteners, but the one I use all the time is-……….

STEVIA (sweetener) - Commonly known as sweet leaf or sugar leaf, STEVIA REBAUDIANA is a widely grown plant. A study has shown it to be a safe and natural, calorie-free sugar substitute. Stevia glycosides are said to be up to 300 times sweeter than sugar. Both the natural zero calorie sweeteners such as Stevia and the artificial ones such as Saccharin has no glycaemic index. They do not raise blood sugar at all. Stevia is a natural zero calorie sweetener and has been proven to be safe. It also appears to help regulate blood sugar levels. With no calories, no sugar and no carbohydrates, stevia's GI score is 0. Stevia was only approved for sale in the EU in 2012, and it was hoped it would prove useful for *diabetics* looking for a naturally derived, low-calorie sweetener. In tests, pure stevia extract has been found to have no effect on blood glucose levels (and may even improve your body's ability to metabolize glucose). In the sense that pure stevia doesn't add calories, affect blood sugar or insulin levels, or contribute to tooth decay, it is a better choice than sugar.

Stevia is a safe and sweet herb which kills stealth and health-robbing bacteria in the stomach, that causes Lyme disease and it kills Lyme disease better than antibiotics.

Replace ½ cup of Stevia in recipes for 1 cup of sugar.

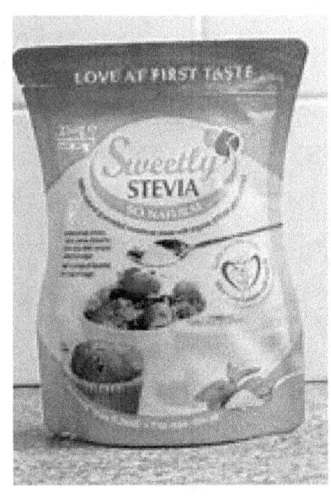 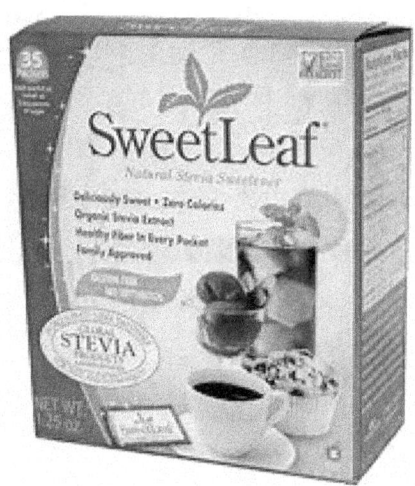

Chapter 7

Changing Your Eating Habits - Step by Step

At this point, it is understood which specific kind of person it takes to productively change their eating habits. We've also learned more about the qualities that one needs in order to look at what you can eat differently. So today, we can now get started with what exactly we are set to accomplish.

Without a doubt, the first step is verifying that you are choosing to change as it can determine your readiness to change your eating habits. You ought to think of choosing to change just like this: no person can truthfully look at what they eat differently without choosing to change. It is literally impossible - that is just how essential this step is.

Choosing to change is also essential if you want to become productive. It will also result with you knowing what you need to do for you and knowing the benefits of healthy eating. The moment you start out choosing to change, you will have a ton to gain - health wise, and absolutely nothing to lose! (or maybe lose some weight).

You also need to continue knowing what is healthy throughout your preparations, and when to change your eating habits. To look at what you eat differently is undoubtedly hard, however knowing what healthy ought to be to help. Plus, choosing to change will help you start boosting vitality, which is clearly important. Boosting vitality ought to help you when you look at what you eat differently now and, in the days, ahead.

Knowing what is healthy also provides more benefits in unique ways outside of changing your eating habits. It should help you know what food you are putting in your mouth and learn what others have gained by eating healthily.

Also knowing what food, you are putting in your mouth is equally important whether you are changing your eating habits or not. So, you should probably consider implementing any method that results in you knowing what foods, the best for you is, to eat.

You may feel ready for changing your eating habits in less than a week once you begin choosing to change, particularly if you know what is healthy.

Typically, 1 week is the approximate period which people plan for getting ready to change by analysing your food journal or diary to find your bad eating habits. Remember these averages when you are calculating your timelines.

Another aspect that is necessary to help you become successful with changing your eating habits is being determined to improve your lifestyle and health. You would not have to narrow in on being determined to improve your lifestyle and health until the second part of your preparations, though certainly do not move past it altogether.

Being able to improve your lifestyle and health ought to assist you to boost energy, which could be beneficial for your preparations. It also encourages you to get into smart routines and get into good eating habits and drinking water often, which in turn encourages you to change your eating habits.

Finally, by choosing to change, knowing what is healthy and being determined to improve your lifestyle and health. It generally requires a week of planning getting truly ready. But, that period ought to go by rapidly.

If you can schedule a fixed date to start your preparation period and mark 1 week later, then it'll lead your brain to see that timeframe as the introductory phase, like setting a goal. At that point, you will be prepared to narrow in on choosing to change, along with knowing what is healthy. Then, you will discover that your entire mind is truly ready to change your eating habits!

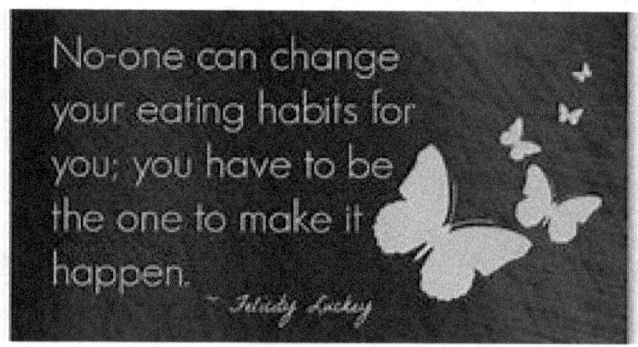

BAD HABITS ARE LIKE A COMFORTABLE BED, EASY TO GET INTO, BUT HARD TO GET OUT OF.

No-one can change your eating habits for you; you have to be the one to make it happen.
~ Felicity Luckey

ONE REASON
PEOPLE RESIST
CHANGE IS
BECAUSE THEY
FOCUS ON
WHAT THEY HAVE
TO GIVE UP,
INSTEAD OF WHAT
THEY HAVE TO
GAIN.

Choices, Chances,
Changes.
You must make a
Choice to take a Chance
or your life will never
Change.

YOU WILL NEVER
CHANGE YOUR LIFE
UNTIL YOU CHANGE
SOMETHING YOU DO
DAILY. THE SECRET
OF YOUR SUCCESS
IS FOUND IN YOUR
DAILY ROUTINE

Chapter 8

Strategies to Changing Your Eating Habits

Changing your eating habits takes a ton out of an individual. Unfortunately, everyone does not really possess what it takes. There are some clear-cut methods that work more powerfully than others to assure that you are unfailingly preparing for your success the best way.

I tell people that you are not going on a 'diet' to change your eating habits but starting a 'healthy eating plan'. Acknowledging this ought to lead you to finally change your eating habits.

Looking at what you eat differently needs one to become committed. So, one that is unchangeable, or has an addiction, might probably not become as successful as they could possibly be. These qualities are inside one who would have said no when approached with the questions asked earlier

Are your eating habits the same as your family (do you all have the same health/weight problems)?

There are qualities for which anybody hoping to change their eating habits must have and being changeable is one of them. The logic behind it is simple. Maintaining a changeable personality is exactly what empowers you to declare yourself as a healthy person after you productively change your eating habits.

Everyone can say that they want to change their eating habits. However, changing is a large step above being obsessive with food. One does not entail a good deal of preparation, and preparation is important to the overall success with the other.

Looking at what you eat differently requires making choices that are right for you and not conforming to others. That may not seem like a big deal, when compared to changing your eating habits, but making choices that are right for you and not conforming to others is very important when you change your eating habits.

Having healthy eating options may be a no-brainer only because it is extremely vital for overall success when you change your eating habits. Having healthy eating options is important while you look at what you eat differently simply due to what is needed.

Thinking and seeing yourself as slim and healthy might also not seem like a big thing, however it certainly is. It is a mind-set, focus on what you want to achieve in the long term. When changing your eating habits, you will need the footwork which you invested time on.

The methods to changing your eating habits help not only the goal of looking at what you eat differently, but each step really comes with a variety of benefits which will complement other aspects of your lifestyle.

It is simple to determine that knowing what you need to do for you is not only an advantage to changing your eating habits, but for life overall. Similarly, boosting vitality is well-known to help other areas of life.

Even boosting energy will become impacting outside of changing your eating habits. Other than being a lifestyle, some people will enjoy how changing their eating habits improves their lifestyle overall.

You might discover when you use these methods to change your eating habits that any existing qualities you had will become significantly enhanced.

Those who are changeable become even more changeable. Similarly, individuals who are beneficial seem even more beneficial. These are among the multiple specific reasons to get started changing your eating habits now!

Chapter 9

Tips to Change Your Eating Habits Successfully

Once you totally commit to changing your eating habits, there are many things that you can try to look at what you eat differently successfully. Here are a handful of tips which will help in changing your eating habits:

> Choosing to change has already been examined in great depth, and that is rather important when you are changing your eating habits. Make sure that you keep your body hydrated and refreshed. Additionally, make it a habit to remember 'you are what you eat' and drink lots of water. This does not only affect changing your eating habits, it affects your lifestyle in general.

➢ You should know that knowing what is healthy is important as well. It may get hard to make happen on your own. So, a great method to foster a feeling of accomplishment as you reach your goals is to keep a journal or food diary and celebrate milestones. This ought to offer you more drive to know what is healthy as you prepare to change your eating habits.

➢ Additionally, know that changing your eating habits needs you to constantly be determined to improve your lifestyle and health. In order to dissuade your mind from becoming discouraged and giving up, it is advisable to remain with a positive attitude and outlook to living a healthy lifestyle.

During the time you reflect these simple tips in your preparation of changing your eating habits, you will discover that you are gaining many benefits. Following are certain benefits which you may recognize as soon as you pursue your commitments to change your eating habits:

> Keep in mind knowing what you need to do for you, will happen much more if you are choosing to change.

> Choosing to change equally permits your body to start knowing the benefits of healthy eating.

> Provided you know what is healthy, it ought to boost vitality.

➢ Additionally, knowing what is healthy helps with knowing what foods you are putting in your mouth.

➢ Through preparing to change your eating habits, and doing some exercise, you can be determined to improve your lifestyle and health and will boost energy because of it.

➢ Being determined to improve your lifestyle and health also will get you into smart routines and setting goals.

Looking at what you eat differently certainly gives a ton of direct benefits, a handful of which we have examined, learning what others have gained by eating healthily, and feeling fit and healthy all the time, all occur when you are choosing to change, knowing what is healthy, and being determined to improve your lifestyle and health.

Looking at what you eat differently involves doing all these things and basking in the benefits that follow. Additionally, following are a handful of additional tips:

> Don't spend money on fancy equipment. 'Know thy self' and what you are putting into your mouth.

> Invest in healthy recipe books or go on-line to find healthy eating plans or try the eating plans in chapter 11 of this book.

> Read about the ingredients in packaged food. If there is a high sugar content - don't buy it or eat it. Like sodas, chocolate, sweets, cakes and biscuits.

The moment you follow the advice included here; you'll be on track to look at what you can eat differently. Keep in mind to allow yourself a week to prepare. Having an adequate period to prepare is vital.

Part of the preparation is clearing out your food cupboards, get rid of the sweets, biscuits and the junk food, so you are not tempted to cheat, which will help your family as well. What the eyes don't see, there is no temptation to have!

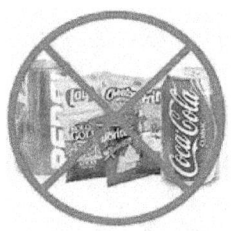

Any tips which would be noted here present a beginning point. The moment reviewing this information, you'll understand what it takes to change your eating habits. Feel free to add your individual observations and develop new instructions to push you to succeed.

Chapter 10

Common Questions About Changing Your Eating Habits

By now, you may be cognizant of the measures you must take to change your eating habits. Say you think of a question which hasn't been addressed, do not fret. Here are three common questions which surface with changing your eating habits:

Is it possible to change your eating habits for free?

For the most part, it is possible to change your eating habits for free. It is pointless to put forth heaps of money preparing to change. Following are a few tips to manage your budget.

➢ Don't spend money on fancy diet groups. 'Know thy self' and what you are putting into your mouth. Each person has different tastes, so go with your own healthy way of eating.

➢ Invest in healthy recipe books or go on-line to find healthy eating plans or read what is healthy in chapter 11.

➢ Read about the ingredients on packaged food. If there is a high sugar content - don't buy it.

Another question which typically comes up when someone is planning to change your eating habits is about the common "rules" to consider while looking at what you eat differently. Following would be certain guidelines to bear in mind:

➢ While choosing to change, remember 'you are what you eat' and drink lots of water. This will keep your body hydrated and refreshed.

➢ Typically, knowing what is healthy is important when looking at what you eat. This will foster a feeling of accomplishment as you reach your goals.

➢ While you narrow in on being determined to improve your lifestyle and health, be sure to remain with a positive attitude, a strong willpower and outlook to living a healthy lifestyle. This will dissuade your mind from becoming discouraged and giving up.

You have taken the initial step toward changing your eating habits by reading more on it. Most likely additional questions may surface and one more way you may benefit yourself is by approaching this goal with a friend or family member that might have similar objectives.

At times a "buddy system" is a great solution while approaching a goal which requires a changeable and beneficial personality. Even though you could ultimately change your eating habits independently, it is advisable to connect with someone on a parallel progression to discuss questions as they surface, like family or friends.

Be mindful to pick like-minded companions and avoid people who may be addictive or unchangeable, as they would drive you away approaching your objectives.

Remember the questions you were asked earlier?

Are your eating habits the same as your family (do you all have the same health/weight problems)?

Are you addicted to junk food? (Are all your meals take-outs?)

Is your body slowing down with aches and pain?

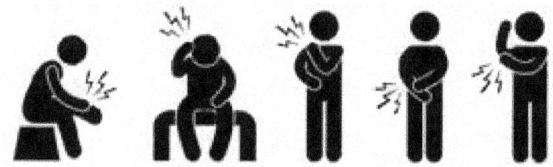

If You have replied yes to the questions, which determined you have the most effective personality to succeed at changing your eating habits. Choose a friend or family member that might also answer yes to these questions as they may also be inclined to succeed at changing their eating habits.

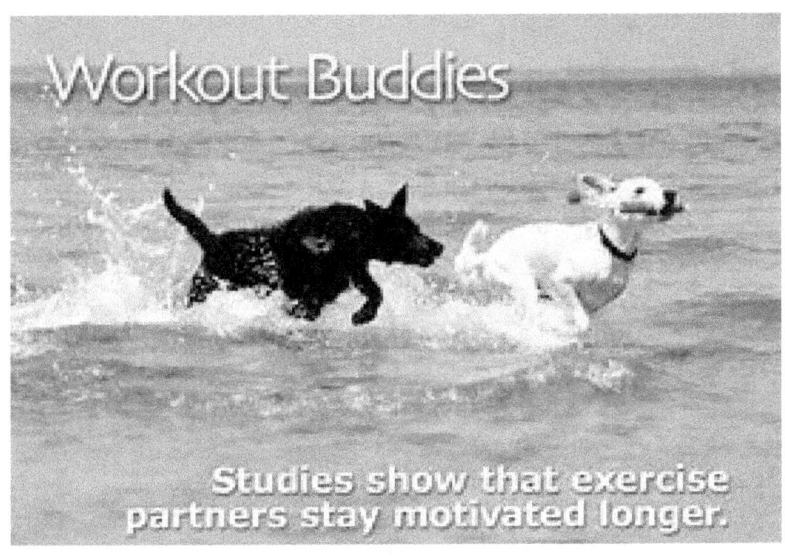

Workout Buddies

Studies show that exercise partners stay motivated longer.

Chapter 11

5 Eating Plans

THE START OF CHANGING YOUR EATING HABITS: -

➤ Drink a cup of hot water and lemon/ginger juice first thing every morning.
➤ During the day drink 1,7 litres of water.
➤ Take multivitamin supplements every day, including (fresh – is best – swallow a small glove of garlic - like a tablet with liquids) or odourless garlic and see suggested list below.

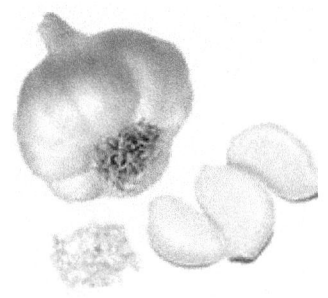

Juice Fast: - Decide on the length (no longer than two or three days) of the fast and take only salads, juices and filtered or distilled Water for two days prior to the fast.

On the morning of the fast, start with a cup of boiling water and lemon juice, then take a glass of either freshly squeezed fruit or vegetable juice mixed 50/50 with water and sip it slowly.

For the duration of the day, have a glass of juice every two hours. You may alternate between fruit and vegetable juices, from the lists below, if you wish, but don't mix the two together.

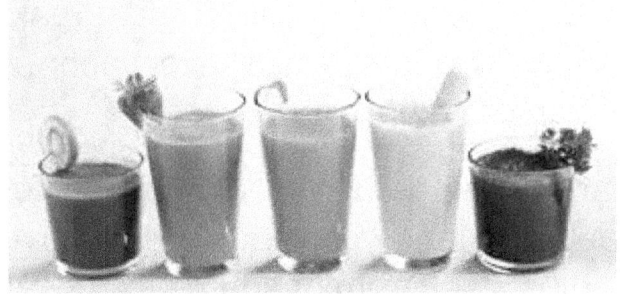

General Fast: - For one week every two months, to help 'detox' your system, only eat food from the foods listed.

Cycle Fasting: - This fasting involves alternate cycles of eating and starvation. This diet can help with weight loss and improve the health of metabolism while protecting the body from a lot of diseases.

It's a type of diet you can activate at the beginning of the season to boost your immune system. Follow for a week at a time.

We are fasting when we sleep, so if we think for a minute, extending that time is no difficulty. Generally, you avoid breakfast, and then you eat lunch after noon, and dinner before 8:00 pm.

Following this path, you are fasting for 16 hours a day, and your body will lose weight and adjust itself from problems.

Suggested ingredients for this diet are:

- Water (fundamental) • Whole grains • Fish • Beans and legumes • Eggs • Cruciferous vegetables (cauliflowers, broccoli, Brussels sprouts) • Probiotics • Berries • Nuts and seeds.

Water, coffee or tea and exercise before noon. Eat between noon and 8 p.m. Then water only and then sleep.

The Raw Food Eating Plan: - it is very simple and gives you lots of energy. As it states absolutely nothing is heated or cooked, you only eat food that is raw and natural. It is fruit, vegetables and nuts. And you only eat when you feel hungry. Eat mixed salads either cut up or grated (even raw potatoes and beetroot).

Carry a bag of mixed nuts to snack on. When you go out with friends to a restaurant, you can feast from the salad bar (if they have one) or order a large salad as your main course. Most places now supply Smoothies so order one to your liking.

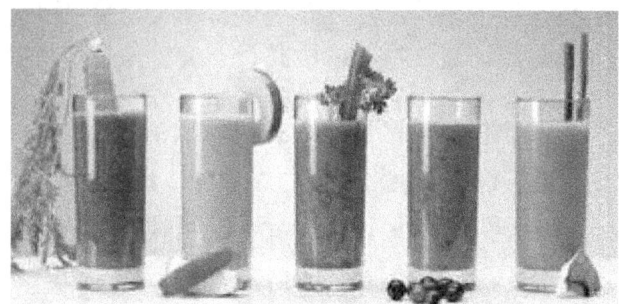

The 3-day Plan - the 3-day plan, is made to lose weight fast. Following this you can lose around 4 or 5 kilograms.

It works in this way: you follow a 3-day meal plan, and then you eat healthy food for the remaining 4 days. Then you repeat it however many times you want until you reach your desired weight. Seems easy, but it's not.

Here are the allowed ingredients:

- Whole-wheat bread (small doses) with peanut butter • Bananas and grapefruit • Carrots • Eggs • Hot dogs • Meat • Tuna • Saltine crackers • Coffee & Tea • Ice cream

Here are the not allowed ingredients:

- Sugar and artificial sweeteners (only Stevia is allowed) • Creamers • Milk • Fruit juices • Oranges • All the rest not included in this list.

Healthy Eating: - To change your eating habits use the Food Lists to spice up what you eat instead. Thinking of the following tips:

> ➢ Remember that *breakfast* is the most important meal of the day, whether you have it first thing in the morning or at 10 a.m. or when you are ready, then lunch 4 or 5 hours later and then dinner 4 or 5 hours later. Meals to be

spread out. A snack, twice a day but only if you feel hungry, it is not important to have if you don't feel like it.

➢ Drink plenty water and herbal teas throughout the day.

➢ Cut out all visible SUGARS (sweets, biscuits, cake, sugar in tea and coffee, use Stevia sweeteners instead, if you must)

➢ Avoid fried foods and pastry in all forms but lightly stir-fried in olive oil is allowed.

➢ For fillers or snacks - Vegetables may be eaten freely, except avocado pears, baked/broad kidney and butter beans. Fruits like grapefruit, lemons, limes, gooseberries, blackberries, raspberries and rhubarb (no sugar added) can be eaten freely. All other fruits 1 or 2 per day.

➤ *Miscellaneous foods* not on the list can be added. Clear soups, meat and yeast extracts, tomato juice, soda water, diet cold drinks and all herbs and spices, but not table salt.

➤ Now for the Naughty List – yes it is difficult to suddenly stop and change how you eat, so have <u>any TWO of these items twice a week</u>: - 1 glass of wine or 2 glasses low alcohol wine, 1 can (350ml) beer or 2 cans Lite beer,   1 tot measure spirits, 1 glass of sherry,   3 toffees,   1 scoop ice-cream or 2 scoops frozen yoghurt   or   sherbet   ice-cream, 1 (50g) small bag of crisps,   1 digestive biscuits   1 small Kit-Kat chocolate, (two fingers) but try to cut out chocolate all together.

➤ The <u>FOODS NOT ALLOWED LIST</u> below is for when you need to detox and improve your health. So, the items can be eaten in moderation, no more than once a day of each food listed *except* the Sugar – that needs to be cut out all together from your eating plan.

➢ There is not a *Meat List* because one should not eat meat when trying to get healthy. But if you do enjoy eating meats, do so only 2 or 3 times a week, but do not eat the fat, cut it off before cooking. Chicken or fish is a healthier alternate.

Junk Food v's Healthy Food

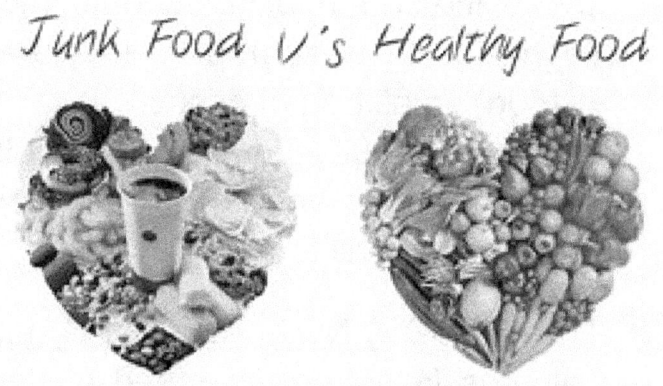

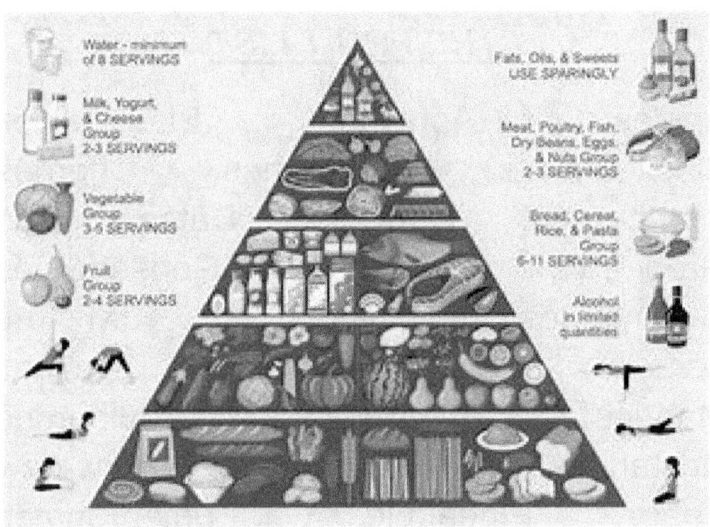

Chapter 12

THE FOOD LISTS

Foods that will increase the body's ability to heal itself, improve your health and cleanse it (help with detoxing). Please remember don't eat anything that is not on these lists:

THE FRUIT LIST

Apples, Apricots, Blackberries, Blackcurrants, Blueberries, Cherries, Cranberries, Currants, Dates, Figs, Grapefruit, Grapes, Gooseberries, Greengages, Guavas, Kiwi fruit, Lemons, Limes, Loganberries, Lychees, Mangos, Melons, Mulberries, Nectarines, Passionfruit, Paw-paw, Pears, Pineapple, Pomegranates, Plums, Prunes, Quinces, Raisins, Raspberries, Redcurrants, Rhubarb,

Sultanas, Strawberries.

THE VEGETABLE LIST

Vegetables to be eaten raw steamed or stir-fried in pure olive oil.

Artichokes, Asparagus, Aubergines, Beans (not lentils), Beetroot, Bean Sprouts, Broccoli, Brussel sprouts, Cabbage, Carrots, Cauliflower, Celery, Chicory, Courgettes, Cucumber, Fennel, Kohlrabi, Leeks, Lettuce (all types), Marrow, Onions, Parsnips, Peas, Peppers, Potatoes, Pumpkin, Radishes, Spring Onions, Sweetcorn, Sweet potatoes, Squashes, Turnips, Watercress, Yams.

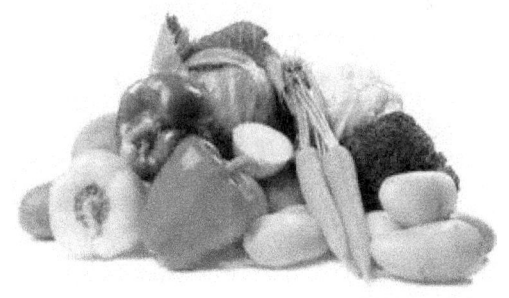

NUTS LIST

Best eaten raw and unsalted.

Almonds, Brazils, Cashews, Chestnuts, Hazelnuts, Macadamia, Pecans, Pine nuts, Pistachio, Walnuts, 'Not allowed Peanuts'

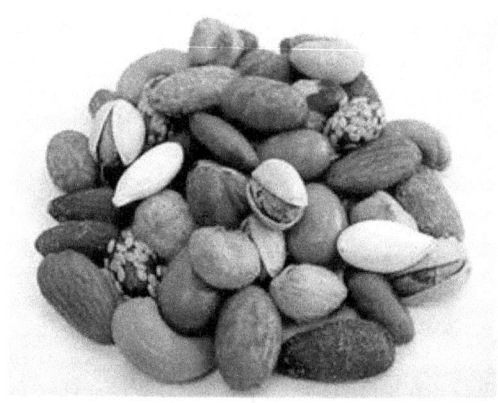

PULSE, SEED, HERB AND SPICE LIST

Alfalfa, Basil, Cardamom pods, Cayenne pepper, Chick peas, Chillies, Chives, Coriander, Dill, Fennel, Ginger, Lemon grass, Marjoram, Mint, Oregano, Parsley, Pepper – ground, Pumpkin seeds, Rosemary, Sage, Sesame seeds, Sunflower seeds, Tarragon, Thyme.

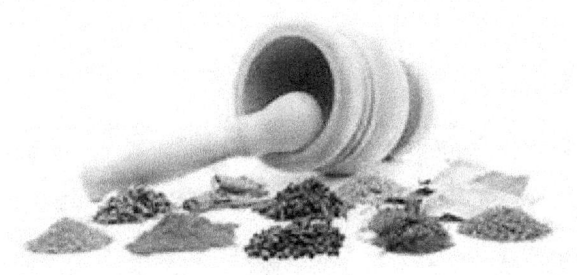

THE FISH LIST

Where possible eat fresh or canned in olive/vegetable oil.

Cod, Crab, Haddock, Herring, Lemon Sole, Lobster, Mackerel, Monkfish, Pilchards, Prawns, Salmon, Sardines, Scampi, Shrimps, Skate, Trout, Tuna.

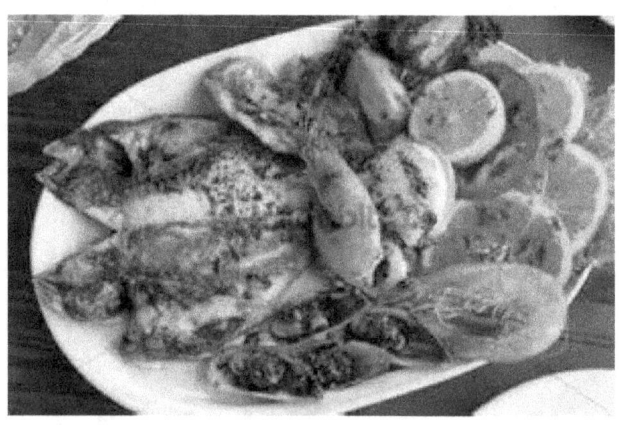

DRINK LIST

Herbal teas (any), Lemon/Ginger, Water.

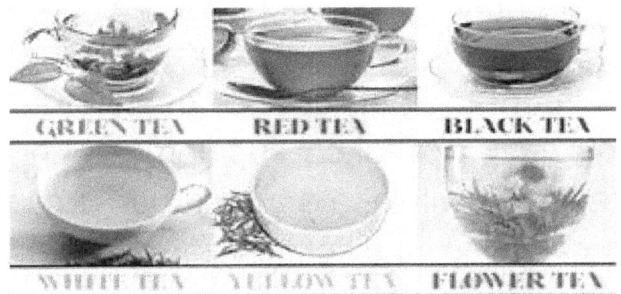

MISCELLANEOUS FOODS

Brown rice (short grain), Balsamic vinegar, Cider vinegar, Grapeseed oil, Mustard grain, Olive oil, Olives (any), Rice cakes – unsalted and no sugar, Seaweed, Sesame oil, Tofu, Walnut oil, Hummus - chickpeas.

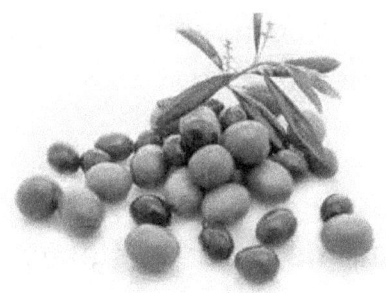

Suggested *VITAMINS LIST*

Please understand that you will not feel the benefits of supplements taking them for a week or so, it is a long-term regiment to keep up. For every year that you have <u>not</u> taken supplements in your lifetime, it will take a month per each year to catch up and feel the true benefits of taking daily supplements.

- ✓ Chromium picolinate – reduces sugar cravings by stabilizing the metabolism of simple carbohydrates (sugar). 1 daily in the a.m.

- ✓ Lecithin capsules – is a fat emulsifier; breaks down fat so it can be removed from your body. 1 at each meal.

- ✓ Spirulina – excellent source of usable protein. Contains needed nutrients and stabilizes blood sugar. 1 between each meal.

- ✓ Vitamin C – a minimum of 1000 mg daily. It is necessary for normal glandular function. It speeds up a slow metabolism, prompting it to burn more calories and good for your immune system. 3 times per day.

- ✓ Vitamin B complex – It is need for proper digestion and gives you energy. 3 times per day.

- ✓ Kelp tablets – is a rich source the B vitamins, minerals and trace elements. (Do not take if you are allergic to iodine). 3 daily.

- ✓ Zinc – not more than 80 mg daily. It enhances the effectiveness of insulin and boosts the immune function. 1 before meals.

Please always remember to read the instruction given with each vitamin. If it states that the dose is the recommended daily allowance RDA – I recommend you take the RDA given and add a couple extra per day to get the full benefit.

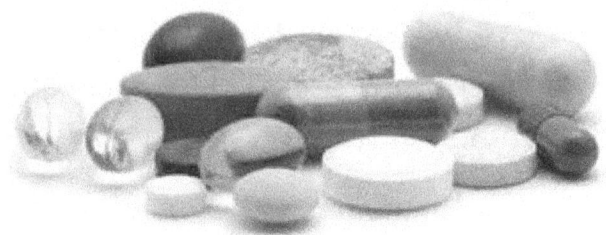

FOODS NOT ALLOWED

Avocados, Bananas, Peanuts = Too much starch and fat

Bread, Rolls = Gluten in wheat flour difficult to digest

Caffeine = Chemical stimulant

Chocolate, Sweets = Too much sugar and fats

Cow's Milk/Cheese etc. = Lactose (milk sugars) difficult to digest

Lentils = Too much gas

Mushrooms = Too much fungus

Oranges, spinach, Tomatoes = Too acidic

Salt = Results in potassium deficiency and water retention

Sugar = The killer! Disturbs blood glucose levels, causing disturbed appetite and energy levels.

All in a neat package: -

Follow these steps to live a Healthy Life.

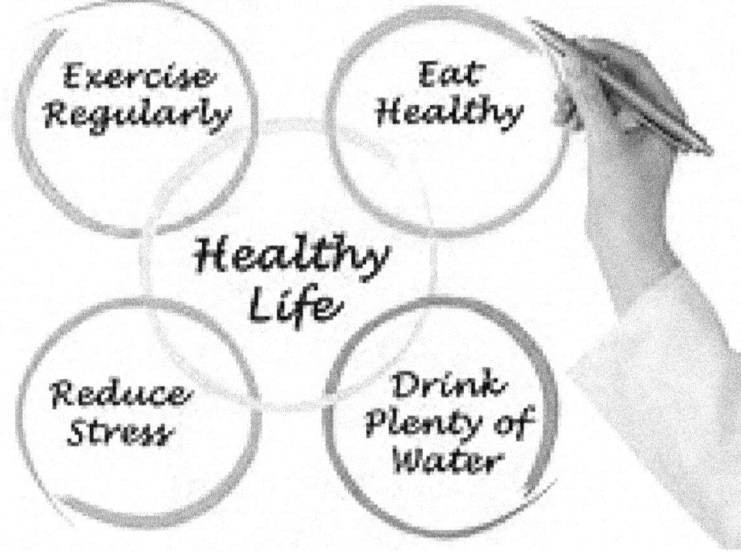

Congratulations on reading this book and I hope you *will* change your eating habits and make it a part of your Life!

None of this is difficult to do in PRACTICAL terms, But psychologically? That's a different matter entirely. First you need to decide whether "Your eating habits are in charge - or YOU are!" ...

If you have enjoyed reading my book can you, please review it?

There is a Colouring Journal and Food Diary to help you change. It is available from Amazon.com books which is part of this series.

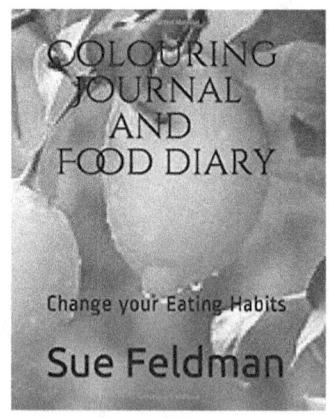

I have two Face Book pages with regards to Health:

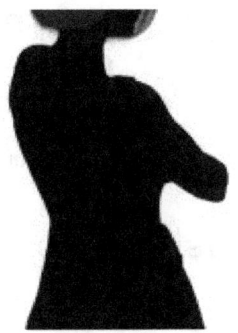

@Diets by Sue

and

@HowToLoseAbdominalFatDietTips

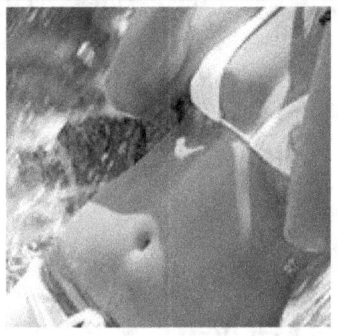

Use and 'like' to get some extra tips and ideas. Please leave a comment and tell your friends on Face book.

I'm just a home-based author with No "big marketing company" behind me, so I highly appreciate your reviews, and it only takes a minute to do.

To submit a review:

1. Just go to Amazon and under the BOOKS category, search this book's title or search my name 'Sue Feldman' to get to the product detail page for this book (or click on the book cover photo).
2. Click '**write a customer review**' in the Customer Review section.
3. Click '**Submit**'

Thank you in advance for submitting.

Sue Feldman (Nut)

Notes to remember: Plan your healthy eating to your likes: Breakfast, lunch, dinner:

_____

_____

_____

_____

_____

_____

_____

_____

_____

_____

_____

www.ingramcontent.com/pod-product-compliance
Lightning Source LLC
Chambersburg PA
CBHW070435290526
45791CB00005B/1980